SURVIVING THE STORM

A Caregiver's Guide to Dementia

Noel R. Bernice

Copyright © 2023 by Noel R. Bernice

All rights are reserved. Except for short quotes used in critical reviews and certain other noncommercial uses allowed by copyright law, no part of this book may be duplicated, copied, or communicated in any way, including by photocopying, recording, or other electronic or mechanical techniques.

TABLE OF CONTENT

INTRODUCTION

CHAPTER ONE

UNDERSTANDING DEMENTIA

What Is Dementia?

Dementia Diagnosis and Treatment

CHAPTER TWO

TAKING CARE OF A LOVED ONE WITH DEMENTIA

Creating a Care Plan

Building a Positive Environment

CHAPTER THREE

ADDRESSING FINANCIAL CHALLENGES

Taking Control of Aggressive and Difficult Behaviors

How to Manage Difficult Emotions

CHAPTER FOUR

PREVENTING BURNOUT

Obtaining Assistance from Experts and Other Caregivers

Giving care: Finding Purpose and Joy

CONCLUSION

INTRODUCTION

As a caregiver for someone living with dementia, you are embarking on a journey that can be both rewarding and mentally draining. You are not alone in your journey since many others have gone before you and have discovered solutions to deal with the challenges that come with this disease.

"Surviving the Storm: A Caregiver's Guide to Dementia" was designed with you in mind to provide you with the resources and assistance you need to travel this path with assurance and delicacy. The advice, tactics, and heartwarming tales in these pages will inspire you to keep going and find pleasure in this lovely if sometimes challenging journey, whether you're just getting started or have been a caregiver for some time.

This book acts as a warm embrace, giving readers the information and encouragement they need to face dementia's storms with grace and tenacity. So let's start this trip toward a better future together as you take a deep breath and hang on to your optimism.

This manual will assist you in comprehending the complexities of dementia and how it impacts your loved one in a compassionate and understanding manner.

You'll discover techniques for controlling behaviors and emotions as well as information on the condition's many phases and the difficulties that each one brings.

This book will provide you with the resources you need to help both yourself and your loved one every step of the journey, from managing stress and preserving your health to finding respite and creating meaningful experiences.

You are an amazing hero and an incredible caregiver. The love and commitment you provide in the face of difficulty are admirable. The message of this book is that you are not alone and that there is hope in the future.

Therefore, maintain your bravery and let "Surviving the Storm: A Caregiver's Guide to Dementia" guide you and your loved one toward a better future.

CHAPTER ONE

UNDERSTANDING DEMENTIA

What Is Dementia?

Dementia is a generic term used to represent a deterioration in cognitive function, which includes memory loss, linguistic difficulties, disorientation, mood swings, and motivational loss. It is a progressive condition that impairs a person's capacity to carry out daily tasks. The majority of cases of dementia in older persons are due to physical abnormalities in the brain, such as damage to nerve cells. It is not a typical aspect of aging, however, and may strike persons as early as their 30s or 40s.

Alzheimer's disease, vascular dementia, Lewy body dementia, frontotemporal dementia, and other conditions fall within the category of dementia. The brain is affected differently by each kind of dementia, which may result in various symptoms. The quality of life of a person with dementia, as well as the lives of their family and friends, may be significantly impacted.

The course of the ailment may be slowed down and quality of life can be increased with early identification and therapy. Along with services like support groups, counseling, and medicine, caregivers play a critical role in providing care and support for dementia patients. With 60 to 80 percent of cases, Alzheimer's disease is the most prevalent kind of dementia.

Memory, language, and reasoning skills gradually deteriorate as a result of this degenerative disorder that affects the brain. It happens when protein accumulations in the brain called plaques and tangles, which harm nerve cells and impair brain function, begin to accumulate. Although there is no known cure for Alzheimer's, there are medicines that may help control the symptoms and delay the disease's development. Particularly in elderly persons, stroke is a major contributor to dementia. When there is a disruption in the blood supply to the brain, brain tissue is harmed, and a stroke results.

Cognitive function may deteriorate as a result, raising the possibility of dementia. Rehabilitation is often used to treat stroke-related dementia to enhance cognitive function and reduce the risk of future strokes.

Abuse of alcohol and other drugs may harm the brain as well, which can result in a reduction in cognitive function and a higher risk of dementia. Wernicke-Korsakoff syndrome, a kind of dementia that impairs memory, coordination, and balance, has been specifically related to chronic excessive drinking.

The risk of stroke and other physical health issues that might hasten the onset of dementia is also increased by substance usage.

Also understand that not everyone with a history of alcohol or drug misuse will get dementia, and not all types of dementia are brought on by these causes. However, it's important to be aware of the risk that drug addiction might result in brain damage and to get treatment if required.

Dementia Diagnosis and Treatment

Dementia is a difficult condition to diagnose and often requires a thorough examination that includes a medical history, physical exam, cognitive and neurological tests, and imaging procedures like MRI or CT scans. The fluid around the brain and spinal cord may sometimes be examined via a lumbar puncture (also known as a spinal tap).

The diagnosis of dementia cannot presently be made with a single test. As opposed to this, a diagnosis is often determined using a pattern of symptoms and the elimination of any other underlying conditions. Sometimes an accurate diagnosis of a particular kind of dementia may only be made after a person has passed away and brain tissue has been analyzed during an autopsy.

Although dementia cannot be cured, some therapies may help control its symptoms

and enhance both the quality of life for those who have the illness and their caretakers.
These remedies may consist of:

Medications:

Memory loss, confusion, and behavioral issues are just a few of the dementia symptoms that may be controlled by several drugs.

The management of dementia symptoms and enhancement of the quality of life for those who have the illness may be greatly aided by medications. Dementia is treated with a variety of drug types, including:

- **Anti-cholinesterase agents:** These drugs, such as galantamine (Razadyne), donepezil (Aricept), and rivastigmine (Exelon), are used to treat mild to severe Alzheimer's disease.

They function by raising the concentrations of acetylcholine, a brain neurotransmitter that aids with memory and thought, in the brain.

- **NMDA receptor blockers:** Memantine (Namenda), among other drugs in this family, is used to treat moderate to severe Alzheimer's disease.

They function by obstructing a particular kind of glutamate receptor in the brain, which aids in preventing harm to brain cells.

- **Antidepressants:** Antidepressant drugs, such as tricyclic antidepressants and selective serotonin reuptake inhibitors (SSRIs), may be used to treat the behavioral and mental symptoms of dementia, such as agitation, anxiety, and sadness.

- **Antipsychotics:** Antipsychotic drugs may be used to treat agitation and psychotic symptoms in dementia patients. Some examples of antipsychotic medications are Risperdal (risperidone) and Zyprexa (olanzapine).

It's vital to understand that these drugs do not treat dementia and do not slow the disease's development. However, they may aid in symptom management and enhance the quality of life for dementia patients and their carers.

When taking any medicine for dementia, it's crucial to work closely with a healthcare professional since there may be adverse effects or drug interactions. As the patient's symptoms and condition evolve, it may be necessary to vary the medication's kind and dose.

Therapy:
Individuals with dementia may enhance their quality of life and keep their independence with the support of cognitive treatment and other forms of therapy.

The quality of life for dementia sufferers and their caretakers may be significantly enhanced by therapy. The following are some typical forms of dementia therapy:

Cognitive therapy may assist people with dementia to keep their cognitive abilities and enhance their memory, language, and problem-solving capabilities. Activities and exercises that stretch the brain and encourage new learning are often used in this sort of treatment.

Treatment for the behavioral and psychological signs and symptoms of dementia, such as agitation, anxiety, and sadness, is behavioral therapy. Techniques for managing symptoms and enhancing general well-being may be used in this kind of treatment, including diversion, stimulation, and relaxation.

- Occupational therapy: Occupational therapy may assist those who have dementia in maintaining their independence and enhancing their capacity to carry out everyday tasks.

The activities and exercises used in this kind of treatment may enhance hand-eye coordination, fine motor skills, and the capacity to carry out daily chores including dressing, eating, and grooming.

- Speech therapy: Speech therapy may help people with dementia become better at speaking and communicating.

This kind of treatment may include speech-improving exercises and activities as well as techniques to enhance communication with loved ones.

- When it comes to assisting people with dementia to reconnect with their memories and emotions, music therapy is a potent instrument.

  Music therapy may entail singing, playing an instrument, or listening to well-known music.

It's necessary to remember that the particular treatment used will depend on the symptoms and demands of the person, and may alter over time as the individual's condition evolves. Working with a healthcare professional and a dementia-specific therapist may assist guarantee that treatment is adapted to the person's unique requirements and objectives.

Lifestyle changes:

Making adjustments to food and exercise, as well as participating in social and mental stimulation, may help control dementia symptoms and enhance general health.

Modifying one's lifestyle may help people with dementia live healthier and more fulfilling lives while controlling their symptoms. Common lifestyle modifications that may aid in managing dementia include:

- **Diet:** Consuming a nutritious diet that is balanced and rich in fruits, vegetables, whole grains, and lean protein will aid with general health and may even decrease the advancement of dementia. According to many research, diets rich in fat and sugar may hasten the onset of dementia.

- **Exercise:** Engaging in regular physical exercises, such as walking, cycling, or swimming, might assist to improve cardiovascular health and perhaps halt the onset of dementia. Mood, sleep, and general well-being may all be enhanced by exercise.

- **Mental stimulation:** Reading, doing puzzles, playing games, or learning a new skill are all mentally stimulating activities that might aid enhance cognitive function and perhaps reduce the advancement of dementia.

- **Socialization** may enhance mood and general well-being, perhaps reduce the onset of dementia, and keep people involved in family, friends, and community activities.

- **Stress management:** Learning effective stress-reduction techniques, like yoga, meditation, or deep breathing, might enhance general health and perhaps delay the onset of dementia.

It's essential to remember that although lifestyle modifications may not be enough to cure dementia, they may be very helpful in controlling symptoms and enhancing both the health and well-being of both those who have the illness and those who care for them. A lifestyle modification should also be personalized and suited to the demands and objectives of the dementia patient.

Support:

For people with dementia and their families, support from family, friends, and professional carers may be both emotionally and practically beneficial.

Caregiving for those with dementia and their families must include support. For those who have dementia and those who care for them, frequent kinds of assistance include:

- Caregiver support groups: Caregiver support groups provide a setting that is safe and encouraging for caregivers to share their experiences, get emotional support, and connect with others who are going through similar difficulties.

Caregiver solace via a brief respite from their caring responsibilities is known as respite care. In-home respite care, adult day care programs, or a brief stay in a nursing home or assisted living facility are a few examples of this.

Home health care services may provide in-home assistance and care for people with dementia, enabling them to stay in their own homes for as long as possible. This might include more complicated medical treatment as well as support with activities of daily life like dressing and washing.

- Memory care facilities: Specialized care facilities created especially for people with dementia. These institutions provide specialized care and assistance for people with dementia, including round-the-clock monitoring, pre-planned activities, and a secure setting.

- Support from professionals: People with dementia and those who care for them may get all-encompassing support and care when they work with a team of healthcare experts, including a doctor, nurse, social worker, and therapist.

Making the appropriate support plan for a person with dementia and their carers requires collaboration with a healthcare physician and other experts.

It's important to collaborate with a healthcare professional to create a tailored treatment plan that takes the person with dementia's unique requirements and objectives into account.

Additionally, early detection and therapy may help the disease's development.

CHAPTER TWO

TAKING CARE OF A LOVED ONE WITH DEMENTIA

Creating a Care Plan

A care plan is a written document outlining the particular care requirements, objectives, and duties for their welfare. A thorough care plan may be created by following the procedures listed below:

Examine the requirements of the person: The person's physical, mental, and emotional condition should be assessed, and any changes that arise over time should be noted. The precise requirements for care and the objectives of the care plan will be determined with the use of this information. Participate the person with dementia in the care-planning process as much as you can. Their perception of autonomy and control may be maintained in this way.

The care team should be identified: it may include family members, friends, and carers with special training. Make sure each individual has their duties well defined before assigning them.

Establish objectives: Specify the objectives for the person with dementia, such as preserving their physical and emotional well-being, guaranteeing their safety, and fostering independence.

Write out your daily schedule: Make a precise itinerary of your daily activities, including your mealtimes, exercise routine, and prescription routines. By doing this, you can be sure the dementia patient is getting the care and attention they need.

Analyze the surroundings: To assure the person's security and comfort, make whatever modifications are required to the home's interior. Putting in grab bars or getting rid of trip hazards are two examples of this.

Prepare for emergencies: Make a strategy for dealing with them, including what to do if someone is lost, about to fall, or otherwise poses a safety risk.

Review and update routinely: As the individual's requirements change over time, the care plan should be periodically reviewed and updated.

The well-being of a loved one with dementia can be guaranteed, and caregivers may provide everyone concerned some peace of mind by developing a thorough care plan.

Building a Positive Environment

For both the dementia sufferer and their caregiver, creating a happy atmosphere for someone with dementia is necessary. Here are some hints to help foster a favorable environment:

Maintain routines:

A person with dementia may feel less stressed and confused if their routine is predictable. Keep your meals, activities, and sleep on a consistent schedule. Maintaining a consistent routine is important for people with dementia because it helps reduce stress and confusion. Here are some ways to help maintain routines:

- **Stick to a schedule:** Having a set schedule for meals, activities, and bedtime can provide structure and stability for the person with dementia.

- **Use reminders:** Visual cues, such as a calendar or a whiteboard, can help remind the person with dementia of what they need to do next.

- **Keep it simple:** Limit the number of activities in a day and make sure they are easy to understand. This can help reduce confusion and stress.

- **Be flexible:** While routines are important, it's also important to be flexible. If the person with dementia is not feeling well or is especially tired, it may be necessary to adjust the schedule.

- **Encourage participation:** Involve the person with dementia in the routine as much as possible. This can help them feel more in control and engaged.

- **Provide structure to leisure time:** Encourage the person with dementia to engage in leisure activities at consistent times throughout the day. This can help provide structure and routine to their leisure time as well.

Encourage independence:
Whenever it is feasible, assist the person with dementia in doing their activities of daily living (ADLs). They'll be able to keep self-control and self-worth thanks to this. Encouraging independence is an important part of creating a positive environment for someone with dementia. Here are some ways to help encourage independence:

- **Offer choices**: Whenever possible, offer choices to the person with dementia. This can help them feel more in control and improve their self-esteem.

- **Encourage ADLs:** Encourage the person with dementia to perform activities of daily living (ADLs) on their own, such as bathing, dressing, and eating. This can enable them to preserve a feeling of authority and autonomy.

- **Use assistive devices:** Assistive devices, such as grab bars and non-slip mats, can help the person with dementia safely perform ADLs on their own.

- **Encourage exercise:** Exercise can help improve the person's physical and mental abilities. Encourage them to engage in physical activity, such as walking or stretching, on their own.

- **Provide opportunities for meaningful activities:** Encourage the person with dementia to engage in meaningful activities, such as hobbies or volunteering, that allow them to use their skills and abilities.

- **Avoid over-protectiveness:** It's important to strike a balance between safety and independence. Over-protectiveness can reduce a person's confidence and self-esteem.

Talk positively:
Refrain from criticizing or speaking negatively. To increase the person's self-confidence and self-esteem, speak to

them positively and compliment them. Using positive language is an important part of creating a positive environment for someone with dementia. The following advice will assist you in speaking positively:

- **Avoid negative language:** Avoid using negative language, such as criticism or blame, when speaking to the person with dementia. This can lead to feelings of frustration and anger.

- **Use affirmations:** Use positive affirmations, such as "I'm proud of you" or "You're doing a great job", to build the person's confidence and self-esteem.

- **Encourage success:** Emphasize the person's successes, no matter how small, and celebrate their accomplishments.

- **Use descriptive language:** Use descriptive language, rather than critical language, to describe the person's behavior. Instead of accusingly stating "You always forget things", try rephrasing it to a more understanding phrase such as "Sometimes you have trouble remembering things".

- **Avoid baby talk:** Avoid using baby talk or speaking to the person with dementia in a condescending manner. This can reduce their sense of dignity and self-esteem.

- **Be patient:** Be patient with the person with dementia and allow them to take their time in completing tasks. Do not cut in when they are speaking or finish their sentences for them.

Create a serene setting:

To create a quiet atmosphere, lessen distractions like loud noise and bright lighting. Providing a serene setting is essential for someone with dementia. Here are some ways to create a calm environment:

- **Reduce noise and distractions:** Minimize noise and distractions, such as loud music or television, in the environment. By doing this, it can aid in decreasing stress and disorientation.

- **Use calming colors:** Use calming colors, such as soft blues and greens, to decorate the environment. This can have a soothing effect on the person with dementia.

- **Provide comfortable furnishings:** Provide comfortable furnishings, such as soft chairs and beds, to create a cozy and relaxed atmosphere.

- **Encourage quiet activities:** Encourage the person with dementia to engage in quiet activities, such as reading or listening to music, which can help them relax.

- **Reduce clutter:** Reduce clutter and keep the environment organized to reduce confusion and anxiety.

- **Use natural light:** Allow natural light into the environment to help improve mood and provide a sense of comfort.

- **Encourage rest:** Encourage the person with dementia to take regular breaks and get adequate rest. Fatigue can increase confusion and anxiety.

Create a comfortable atmosphere by surrounding the individual with familiar items and images. This may calm you and make you feel less anxious. Creating a familiar environment can help improve the quality of life for someone with dementia.

Here are some ways to create a familiar environment:

- **Use familiar objects and items:** Surround the person with familiar objects, such as photos, furniture, and keepsakes, to help stimulate their memory and create a sense of comfort.

- **Create a familiar routine:** Establish a familiar routine, including regular meals and activities, to provide a sense of stability and comfort.

- **Encourage familiar activities:** Encourage the person with dementia to engage in familiar activities, such as gardening or cooking, that they used to enjoy.

- **Use familiar music:** Play familiar music, such as favorite songs or oldies, to help stimulate memories and create a sense of comfort.

- **Use familiar scents:** Use familiar scents, such as perfumes or cooking spices, to help stimulate memories and create a sense of comfort.

- **Provide a familiar setting:** Provide a familiar setting, such as a favorite room or outdoor area, where the person can relax and feel at ease.

Encourage sociability by getting the dementia patient involved in family and friend activities, their mood and general well-being may be enhanced as a result. Encouraging socialization is an important part of creating a positive environment for someone with dementia. Here are some tips to help encourage socialization:

- **Organize social activities:** Organize social activities, such as group outings or parties, to provide opportunities for the person with dementia to interact with others.

- **Encourage participation in group activities:** Encourage the person with dementia to participate in group activities, such as group games or discussions, to help build their confidence and social skills.

- **Provide opportunities for one-on-one interaction:** Provide opportunities for one-on-one interaction, such as visits from friends or family, to help the person with dementia feel connected and supported.

- **Encourage communication:** Encourage the person with dementia to communicate with others, even if it is just a simple conversation or exchange of ideas.

- **Promote physical touch:** Promote physical touch, such as holding hands or giving hugs, to help build a sense of comfort and connection.

- **Use technology:** Use technology, such as video calls or virtual meetings, to allow the person with dementia to stay connected with others even if they are unable to physically meet.

Use humor: Laughter is a wonderful stress reliever and may help to foster a happy atmosphere. Encourage the person with dementia to laugh at commonplace events by trying to discover the comedy in them. The use of humor can play an important role in creating a positive environment for someone with dementia. Here are some ways to incorporate humor into caregiving:

- **Share jokes and funny stories:** Share jokes and funny stories with the person with dementia to help lighten the mood and improve their emotional well-being.

- **Use humor in daily activities:** Use humor in daily activities, such as making silly faces or telling silly jokes, to help the person with dementia relax and have fun.

- **Encourage laughter:** Encourage the person with dementia to laugh by engaging in activities that they find funny, such as watching comedies or listening to funny podcasts.

- **Create a light-hearted atmosphere:** Create a light-hearted atmosphere by adding decorations, such as funny posters or whimsical figurines, to the environment.

- **Play games with humor:** Play games with the person with dementia that are fun and light-hearted, such as charades or silly guessing games.

- **Celebrate special events with humor:** Celebrate special events, such as birthdays or holidays, with humor by telling jokes or singing silly songs.

The quality of life for the dementia patient and their caregiver may be enhanced by using these suggestions to create a happy atmosphere.

CHAPTER THREE

ADDRESSING FINANCIAL CHALLENGES

Caring for someone with dementia can come with significant financial challenges. Here are some steps that can help address these challenges:

- **Research financial assistance programs:** Research financial assistance programs, such as Medicaid or the Alzheimer's Association, that can provide financial help for individuals with dementia and their caregivers.

- **Create a budget:** Create a budget to track expenses and identify areas where costs can be reduced.

- **Plan for long-term care:** Plan for long-term care, such as nursing home or in-home care, and estimate the associated costs. Consider purchasing long-term care insurance to help cover these costs.

- **Consider alternative living arrangements:** Consider alternative living arrangements, such as a shared living situation, that can be more affordable and provide support for both the person with dementia and the caregiver.

- **Utilize community resources:** Utilize community resources, such as local support groups, to find resources and services that can help reduce the financial burden of caregiving.

- **Seek legal and financial advice:** Seek legal and financial advice from a qualified attorney or financial advisor to help ensure that the person with dementia's assets is protected and used in the best way possible.

By taking these steps, you can help address financial challenges and ensure that the person with dementia receives the care and support they need.

Taking Control of Aggressive and Difficult Behaviors

Dementia can sometimes cause aggressive and difficult behaviors in individuals with the condition. Below are some strategies to help manage these behaviors:

- **Identify triggers:** Identify what triggers the aggressive or difficult behaviors, such as changes in routine or physical discomfort, and try to avoid or minimize these triggers.

- **Use positive reinforcement:** Use positive reinforcement, such as praise or treats, to encourage desired behaviors and discourage aggressive or difficult behaviors.

- **Provide a calm environment:** Provide a calm and supportive environment, such as a quiet room or comfortable seating, to help reduce stress and anxiety.

- **Redirect attention:** Redirect the person with dementia's attention to a different activity or task when they become agitated or aggressive.

- **Avoid confrontations:** Avoid confrontations and use a calm and soothing tone of voice when speaking to a person with dementia.

- **Seek professional help:** If aggressive or difficult behaviors become unmanageable, seek professional help from a behavioral specialist or therapist.

How to Manage Difficult Emotions

Caring for someone with dementia can evoke difficult emotions, such as frustration, sadness, or stress. Here are some suggestions for controlling these feelings:

Practice self-care: Practice self-care by engaging in activities you enjoy, such as exercise or hobbies, to help reduce stress and improve your mood. Practicing self-care is crucial for managing the emotional demands of caregiving. Below are some specific strategies for engaging in self-care:

- **Engage in physical activity:** Engage in physical activity, such as exercise or yoga, to help reduce stress and improve your physical and emotional well-being.

- **Take breaks:** Take breaks from caregiving responsibilities, such as by taking a walk, reading a book, or engaging in a hobby, to help reduce stress and improve your overall mood.

- **Eat a balanced diet:** Eat a balanced diet that includes plenty of fruits, vegetables, and whole grains to help improve your physical and emotional health.

- **Get enough sleep:** Make sure you are getting enough sleep each night to help reduce stress and improve your overall mood.

- **Connect with others:** Connect with friends, family, or support groups to help manage the emotional demands of caregiving.

- **Seek professional help:** Consider seeking help from a therapist or counselor to address any emotional challenges you may be facing.

Seek support: Seek support from family, friends, or support groups to help cope with the emotional demands of caregiving.

Get help from professionals: Consider seeking help from a therapist or counselor to address any emotional challenges you may be facing.

Practice relaxation techniques: Practice relaxation techniques, such as deep breathing or meditation, to help manage stress and improve your overall emotional well-being. Stress management and unpleasant emotions may both benefit from relaxation practices. You might try the following methods:

- **Deep breathing:** Pay attention to taking long, steady breaths with your mouth open and your nose closed. This may aid in mental relaxation and stress reduction. To relieve tension and lessen stress, alternate between tensing and relaxing various muscle groups in your body.

  Focusing on the present moment and your breath can help you to practice mindfulness meditation. This may aid in lowering stress and enhancing mental health.

- **Visualization:** To assist quiet the mind and lessen tension, close your eyes and picture a serene environment, such a beach or a forest.

- **Yoga:** Engage in mild stretching or yoga to help lower stress and enhance your physical and mental wellbeing.

- Guided imagery: To help you relax and cope with stress, listen to a guided imagery tape.

Set realistic goals: Set realistic goals for caregiving and break tasks down into manageable steps to help reduce stress and avoid burnout.

Find moments of joy: Make time to find moments of joy and laughter with the person with dementia, such as playing games or going for a walk.

CHAPTER FOUR

PREVENTING BURNOUT

Prioritizing self-care and establishing boundaries Setting limits and making yourself a priority are crucial steps in handling the emotional demands of caring. Here are some guidelines for making self-care a priority and setting boundaries:

- **Make time for self-care:** Schedule self-care activities like exercise or hobbies to help you relax and feel better overall. To safeguard your time and energy for your caregiving obligations, set limitations and boundaries with friends and family.

- **Seek assistance:** To lighten the load of caregiving duties, think about asking for assistance from family, friends, or support groups.

- **Delegate duties:** Assist in lightening a load of caregiving obligations by assigning tasks, such as grocery shopping or housework, to other family members or friends.

- **Get assistance:** To help you handle the emotional demands of caring, consider seeking assistance from a therapist, counselor, or support group.

- **Say no:** Develop the skill to decline extra obligations and commitments that can cause stress and interfere with your ability to give self-care the priority it deserves.

While providing dementia care, you may lessen stress and enhance your general emotional well-being by emphasizing self-care and setting boundaries.

Obtaining Assistance from Experts and Other Caregivers

To make sure you are giving your loved one the best care possible, getting assistance from professionals and other caregivers is a crucial step. You may get the help and information you need to make the caregiving journey effective by exploring the resources that are available and making connections with professionals and other carers.

- **Identify Your Needs:** Before you start looking for assistance, it's critical to identify the kind of support you need. Think about the particular difficulties you are experiencing, such as time management difficulties, mental and physical distress, and any other matters that need care.

- **Contact Local Organizations:** Caregiver assistance is available from several local organizations and initiatives. Speak with nearby businesses that provide assistance and support to carers. These organizations can tell you about support groups, useful resources, and caring services.

- **Connect with Experts:** Get in touch with professionals in the caregiving industry to find out more about the services and resources that are available. They can advise you on how to take the best possible care of your loved one.

- **Join an Online Support Group** There are several Online Support Groups devoted to Caregivers, so consider joining one. You may meet other carers who are dealing with the same difficulties by attending a support group. You may share your experiences and learn from one another.

- **Use Community Resources:** Caregivers may use a variety of community resources. Utilize these tools and resources to assist in caring for your loved one.

- Join a Caregiver Network: Being a part of a caregiver network has certain advantages. You may interact with other caregivers via a network like this and exchange information, counsel, and support.

Giving care: Finding Purpose and Joy

Caregiving can be a rewarding but also challenging experience, it's important to find purpose and joy in it. The following advice might be helpful:

Focus on the positive: While caregiving can be demanding, try to focus on the positive aspects of your relationship with your loved one and the opportunity to help. Maintain a healthy balance: Make time for yourself and prioritize self-care to avoid burnout.

Find meaning in your role: Consider how your caregiving is making a difference in your loved one's life and how it contributes to your sense of purpose and fulfillment.

Celebrate small victories: Recognize and celebrate small victories, like improved health or enjoyable activity.

Remember to take care of yourself and find joy in the journey, this can make all the difference in the caregiving experience.

CONCLUSION

In conclusion, "Surviving the Storm: A Caregiver's Guide to Dementia" provides a comprehensive and compassionate guide for anyone who is caring for a loved one with dementia. Through this book, you have learned about the various stages of dementia and the challenges that come with each stage. You have also been provided with practical tips and strategies to help you manage your own stress and maintain a healthy balance while providing care.

Above all, the book has emphasized the importance of self-care and finding joy in the caregiving journey. Remember, dementia is a storm that can be difficult to navigate, but with the right support, knowledge, and a positive outlook, you can weather it with grace and compassion. Caring for a loved one with dementia is a journey that requires patience, understanding, and resilience. Take care of yourself, and ask for help from others when you need it. You are not alone.

www.ingramcontent.com/pod-product-compliance
Lightning Source LLC
Chambersburg PA
CBHW050331220526
45465CB00018B/1870